GUIDE TO SOLVE
SEX PROBLEMS
(WITH 60 POSTURES)

R.K. Pal

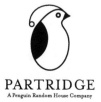

PARTRIDGE
A Penguin Random House Company

To order additional copies of this book, contact
Partridge India
000 800 10062 62
www.partridgepublishing.com/india
orders.india@partridgepublishing.com

DEDICATION

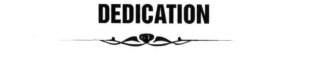

This Comprehensive and dictionary type Book, acts as a Sex Stimulator-cum-Booster, is dedicated to those, who

1. Make use of sex properly in day-to-day activities for the betterment of themselves and our society.

2. Make sincere attempts to satisfy the partner equally without playing selfish game during sexual activities.

3. Educate others, who have wrong concepts / believes on sexual matters with explanation.

4. Help society to prevent sexual offences like molestation / rape etc.

5. Restrict themselves during their own sexual activities so that others in this mixed society are not got excited.

* Good Wisher

*Note: I Prefer to be considered me as your Good Wisher instead of Author.

An Appeal to my Couple Readers:

To my male couple:

1. Do not treat sex organs of your wife as your personal use-cum-property and utilize them with her consent only directly / indirectly. Thus do not play selfish game in sex play.

2. Being active player on sex game, it becomes <u>Prime Duty and Responsibility of husband</u> to make sure that his partner also get 100% sex satisfaction in sex play along with him. For it husband has to study her sex organs as response of sex organs varies from person to person and sometimes it may take 6 months. So investigate it silently with patience.

3. Do not play sex game, when you / both of you are in worry-cum-mental tension. Because this tension will definitely will re-appear automatically during sex play. Ultimately it will make permanent damage on both of your sex organs, which may lead to break down your marriage too. Thus make sure that <u>both of your minds are completely free during sex play.</u>

To my female couple:

1. Open up your mind to husband and do not feel shy to express yourself. If you do not say, how husband will be able to understand you? Thus you must make yourself completely free during sex play.

2. You are passive (not active) player in sex game. Remember that couple are complementary to each other in sex game too. In that case if you do not co-operate with your husband, yourself will not get 100% sex satisfaction but husband will get 100% sex satisfaction being active player in sex game. But in the long run husband will loose attraction towards you, which may lead to break down your marriage too. Thus it is <u>Prime Duty and Responsibility of wife</u> to co-operate husband in all respects.

INDEX ON CHAPTER WISE

INDEX ON MATTER WISE

(Serves as a Dictionary)

.

CHAPTER I

GENERAL KNOWLEDGE ON SEX MATTERS

AT A GLANCE:

1. The following matters may be useful to solve your sex problems:

    (A) General knowledge on Sex Matters (Page: 1)

    (B) Common sex related problems of male and female (Page: 98)

    (C) Pre-love play, Intercourse (Coitus), Orgasm and Masturbation (Page: 45)

    (D) Details of Intercourse with 60 Postures (Page: 55)

    (E) General knowledge on Male Sex Organs (Page: 18)
         (Important for all males)

(F) General knowledge on Female Sex Organs
     & Indirect Sex Organs (Page: 22 & 25)
     (Important for all males)

(G) Penis (Page: 29)
     (Important for all males)

(H) Menstruation cycle / Menses (Page: 39)
     (Important for all females)

(I) Pregnancy, Child birth (Page: 84)
     (Important for all females)

2. Couple must study and understand the
   characteristic behavior and function of own
   as well as partner's sexual parts. They then
   co-operate each other and act accordingly during
   sex play. It is very much necessary to maintain
   the family peace and to make their marriage life
   successful and enjoyable in all respects.

3. Remember that sex is not only for intercourse
   or enjoyment purpose. Sex is a source of life
   (like the sun is called as a source of life). Thus
   be very careful during sex game. If you are in
   tense or mind is not stabilized due to some
   reasons, then please do not go for sex. It will
   not reduce your tense, but it will make harmful
   even will damage you sexual parts. If you do sex
   repeatedly in disturbed mind condition, then this
   damage also carry forward. Then one day this
   damage will be so great, which may even lead to

divorce. Thus make sure that both of your minds are completely FREE during sex play.

4. Keep on changing the intercourse posture now and then in order to stimulate and boost the sex desire and keep your same sex partner attractive and interesting forever.

What inspires me to make this book?

After discussion with various aged people (male and female)of various societies on sex matters including social customs, I observe mainly <u>three short-comes</u> namely:

1. People get bored on sex life after 2/3 years of marriage. Because same types of intercourse posture (may be 1, 2 or 3) are being used every time. Similarly if we take same types of food daily, we get fed up. Thus we keep on changing our menu daily to change our food test. Here also our types of intercourse postures are required to change frequently to keep our sex alive as well as attractive till the last. Then our attraction on intercourse will not get fed. Moreover it will keep on attractive your same sex partner till last.

Thus in this book, <u>60 types of intercourse postures</u> are mentioned. In each and every intercourse posture, the following points are mentioned, when applicable:

(a) Any advantage/disadvantage on that posture?

(b) Advisable during pregnancy period?

(c) Suitable for new couple?

(d) Suitable for Slag penis holder (whose penis gets erected in excitement, but does not hold stiffness for longer period due to some reasons)?

2. People are not freely open minded on sex matters. Senior people do not guide, even say anything to juniors on this matters. Thus People keep carry on a lot of wrong thoughts / ill-concepts / unwanted fear in the name of god or society.

As for examples:

A. Some females think that during menses period she remain "dirty" and thus not allowed to take part in any social works. Even some females think that menses is a god-given punishment to female. I observe that most of females are not at-all aware of her own physics and thus not able to maintain her own health. Thus they do not know why menses occurs, what precautionary measures to be taken during this period and how to reduce the pain, if occurs.

B. Some males think that masturbation is a sin and consists of lot of blood. He further thinks that since he could not avoid masturbation due to some reasons, his health going down day-by-day.

C. It is quite natural that Younger have curiosity on sex matters such as why penis get erected during excitement only, not normal time? Why urine and semen can not be possible to pass through penis together at a time? Why breast of male do not grow bigger at puberty? What's menses and why female discharges blood during menses? Is also female discharge liquid at the peak point of excitement like male? etc. etc.

All these sex quarries are discussed separately in the CHAPTER I (General knowledge on sex matters: page-1), CHAPTER IV (Menstruation cycle / Menses: page-39) & CHAPTER VIII (Common sex related problems of male & female:page-98).

3. In this modern nuclear competitive life, people do not have time to pay attention to learn on sex, though wanted to play big roll on it. Lot of books on sex are available in market. Their main purpose is to attach the decorated colored sexy pictures to excite people and make money.

Off-course a few good books on sex are also available but they are too lengthy and with medical words, which is not easy to understand for common people.

This book is prepared as a Comprehensive and dictionary type book as well as a Sex Stimulator-cum-Booster.

Now it is up to the Readers how much <u>they can make useful for their goodness</u>.

What is the specialty of this Book?

1. To Understand the importance of sex in our daily life in all respects.

2. Female should be aware of her own physics so that she can maintain her own health and the development of offspring, known as an "Embryo"or "Fetus"in her uterus during pregnancy. Thus the "<u>CHAPER VII (Pregnancy, child birth & status of new born child: page</u>-84) is elaborated little more.

3. To Enjoy sex with partner without playing selfish game and must take the responsibility to satisfy the sex partner 100%, not partially. Please note that if female does not satisfy fully in sex play, it has side effects like not getting sleep or headaches etc. and later on turns into serious

psychiatric problem. Thus the "CHAPTER I (General knowledge on sex: page-1) & CHAPTER V (Pre-love play, Intercourse (Coitus), Orgasm and Masturbation: page-45) is elaborated little more.

4. To Keep sex attraction alive till end of life by using different types of intercourse postures. Thus the "CHAPTER VI (Intercourse with 60 Postures: page-55) is elaborated little more.

5. All matters are discussed on practical real life basis considering our mixed society.

6. All matters are discussed in short, not in details. Thus it can be called as Short Note on sex matters.

7. All matters are discussed in simple way with line sketches / diagrams so that readers can understand easily, follow them and it will save the valuable time.

8. All books have only one INDEX. But this book has two INDEX, One on Chapter wise as usual. Other one is prepared on matters / subjects wise. It will serve as a dictionary. It will also save your valuable time.

**How to solve sex problems??

1. Person should have overhaul general idea on all important parts, organs of various systems of human body.

2. Then they must have little more knowledge on sex organs of own as well as partner too.
(Note: Some one may have sound knowledge on sex organs, but no idea on other systems due to which suffering and mind got disturbed. In this unstable mind, sex problems could not be solved. Even during headache sex could not be enjoyed).

3. The most important factor to solve the sex problems is <u>CO-OPERATION</u>, because sex is a combination of dual act and dual operation. It is the vital factor, by which most of sex problems will be dissolved itself automatically. If still pending, co-operation will definitely reduce the sex problems to a great extend.

4. Sometimes sex problems may be due to either physical deficiency or mental dis-balance. For physical deficiency, medical treatment necessary where as for mental problems, counseling must. As per medical report, cases of mental problems is much more (about 80%) than that of physical deficiency.

A. Human Body in short:

Human body is nothing but a GREAT & UNIQUE computer but having LIFE & MOTION.

1. Body is to be maintained properly and carefully.

2. Various systems of human body work continuously 24 hours with its own, even during sleeping like breathing, digestion etc.

3. Some system takes precautionary measure, if un-wanted things happened. If a fly sits on body, hands will reach that place and drive the fly away, even during sleep time too.

4. Most of systems (not all) have dual organs such as two hands, two legs, two eyes, two nasal holes etc. Even brain has two chambers. Thus if one organ gets damaged due to some reasons, other one will take charge automatically.

5. One more precautionary measure in our body: Generally most of our blood veins, which supply nursing food to the various cells, are kept behind the organs so that veins do not get damaged easily at first instant.

B. Sex Organs in short:
See Page: 18

What is sex?

1. When someone utter "sex", first impression comes in our mind as intercourse or something like that – is it not?
   Second thought is that it means by which we differentiate a person whether Male or Female.

2. But in practical field, sex is a source of life (like sun is called as a source of life).

3. Sex is an inspiration of life, which makes our life smooth, enjoyable, happy and builds strength in mind to fight against any odds, sorrow and also helps to digest the past unwarranted incidents.

4. Sex makes life rolling with hopes. Other way it can be called as booster for the momentum of life. That is why, after deep sorrow also person again start daily routine jobs.

Note: Difference in physical sex activities:

There is a deference between male and female in the field of sex activities. In sex activities, male has to take active part, where as female remains in passive action. Thus if male is in sorrow mode, he can not take active part in sex play as his penis will not erect at-all, where as female can take part in sex play though she may feel uneasy or pain.

Due to this physical difference, you will be astonished to know that <u>50 to 60% female do not get complete satisfaction</u> during each time intercourse.

How to confirm that female too get 100% satisfaction (orgasm) along with male in the intercourse?

(A) Indications of satisfaction during intercourse:

i)   Internal parts of female vagina will discharge so much liquid that male will feel it and due to this discharge his penis will become too loose inside vagina and he will hear some peculiar sound coming from vagina during penis movement.

ii) Female may behave abnormally like shaking her some sexual parts abnormally or abnormal sound coming from her mouth. These will be happened without her sense.

iii) Female may hold grip on male harder at the rate of getting excitement. Hardest grip, when more excitement.

(B). Indications of satisfaction at the end of intercourse:

i)   Male will feel that his penis is getting compressed and released several times by vagina wall and thereafter stopped.

ii) Female's abnormal behavior will stopped.

iii) Female will loosen the grip on male.

iv) Female will feel deep sleep immediately after intercourse.

Why penis of male erected and enlarged, only when gets sexually excited?

See the CHAPTER II (A): Sl. No. 2 (corpus cavernosum) of MALE SEX ORGANS (Page: 18) & CHAPTER III of Erection of penis (Page:12 & 30). Body / Shaft of penis consists of 3 internal chambers, made up of special and sponge-like erectile tissue. This tissue contains thousands of large spaces that get filled with blood, when male is excited and that blood could not come out. Thus penis gets erected , enlarged and rigid.

Why penis of male does not come out of vagina during return stroke of the intercourse?

It is due to peculiar shape of Glans of penis (Page:20 & 30). Front portion of Glans is tapper with smaller diameter at the tip(head), which enters vagina at-first. So front portion will help penis to penetrate inside vagina smoothly and easily. But rear portion of Glans is bigger diameter and probe-like shape with slot. Thus the rear portion will resist penis to come out of vagina easily during return stroke of intercourse.

Why breast of male does not grow bigger at puberty like female?

See the CHAPTER II (C): INDIRECT SEX ORGAN: Breast (Page: 25).

Breast tissue of both male and female consists of tubular structure, known as "Ducts".

At puberty female's ovaries produce female hormones, ie, "Estrogen", which causes the ducts to grow and also milk glands ,ie, "Lobules" to develop at end of ducts. Amount of fat and connective tissue in breast also increases as female reaches puberty. These lobules can produce milk, when they receive the appropriate hormonal stimulation. Breast ducts transfer milk from lobules out to nipples and then milk exits from nipples while sucking.

Please note that here is the deference for male. Male hormones, ie, "Testosterone" suppress the growth of breast tissue and lobules. This is the reason that male breast does not grow at puberty.

What's menses and why female discharges blood during menses?

Menses indicate that no pregnancy occurred. As per menstrual circle of a female (generally age of 12 to 50), one egg ,ie, ova from ovaries get matured for production of new born once in a month, provided ova gets chance to meet the able sperm of male. If ova meets the sperm, pregnancy occurred and no menses thereafter. If ova could not meet the sperm, then only menses started for the following reason:

See the CHAPTER II (B): Sl. No. 7 (Uterus / Womb) of FEMALE SEX ORGANS (Page: 22) . Inner layer of uterus is made of blood and known as 'Endometrium". This layer grows thicker by discharge of one type of hormone (FSH). If no pregnancy is occurred, then this blood layer only comes out through vagina as menses during menses period.

How to increase the duration of sexual intercourse in order to avoid pre-mature ejaculation, ie, discharge and able to enjoy the sex maximum time?

Here I will tell you a new technique, by which you can solve this great and general problem, if there is no physical deficiency.

Since it is a common and nature phenomena that female gets excited at slower rate than male, thus female does not get proper satisfaction. Now we should do something to overcome this deficiency. Thus we have to make sure that female gets orgasm faster and at the same time male gets it later. There are the following three remedies to overcome this deficiency:

1. Before starting of actual intercourse, pre-love play is to be continued for longer period so that excitement of female reaches near orgasm.

2. Before inserting the penis in to vagina, a little oil, preferable coconut oil, is to be put on the head of penis / glans. This oil will be utilized as lubrication. Thus it will reduce the friction between the penis and the inside wall of vagina. Once the friction is reduced, then excitement feeling also will be reduced. Ultimately duration of intercourse time will be increased.
   Notes: During excitement female discharges various types of secretions. These secretions are

also act as lubrication. Since female gets excited at slower rate than male, thus <u>additional oil on penis will help for faster lubrication.</u>

3. During intercourse time, Just little before discharge of semen, male has to do two things:

   (A) To divert his attention of mind to other matter so that his excitement gets reduced.

   (B) To hold his breathing as much as possible.

It is not an easy job. It <u>requires some practice</u>; then only he will be able to control his discharge of semen as and when he wants.

Is female discharge at orgasm like male? How male & female enjoy orgasm?

No, female do not discharge at orgasm. Male enjoys orgasm (ie, pleasure of intercourse) by discharging semen, where as female enjoys it by vaginal contraction.

Why female should clean the vagina with soap-water at-least once in a day?

During excitement female discharges various types of secretions.

(A) In addition of lubrication property, these secretions have a <u>special of smelling, which makes the male attracted and sexually excited.</u>

(B) If these secretions remain inside the vagina for longer period, they get spoiled and cause for itching.

Thus female must make habit to clean the inside of vagina periodically and at-least once in a day with soap-water.

Why Viagra is not recommended for erection of penis or as a treatment for impotency?

Please note that now-a-days male is using a drug <u>sildenafil citrate</u> for erection of penis for longer period or as a treatment for impotency. It is sold under the brand name Viagra. Primary drawback of Viagra is that it works about an hour after it is taken. More over it is harmful for diabetes, high blood pressure etc. Thus it is recommended to use it after consultation with Doctor only.

CHAPTER II

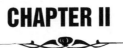

GENERAL KNOWLEDGE ON SEX ORGANS

At first we must have General knowledge on our sex organs to understand them. We have to look at new born's Genital (sex organ: penis / vagina) to confirm whether new born is male or female.

However short description are given on main parts only.

(A) MALE SEX ORGANS:

Short description of male sex organs:

The main male sex organs are as follows:

1. Penis
2. Corpus cavernosum (2 nos.)
3. Corpus spongiosum
4. Foreskin of Glans
5. Glans
6. Scrotum
7. Testicle (2 nos.)
8. Epididymis (2 nos.)

9. Urinary bladder
10. Prostate gland
11. Urethra

1. **Penis**: Most active and sensitive sex organ of male during intercourse period. Size in India: When un-excited, 3 to 4 inches in length and 2 to 3 inches in circumstance. But when excited (erected), size becomes larger and its muscles become very rigid. Then it will be 5 to 9 inches in length and 2.5 to 4 inches in circumstance. But it differs in various individuals of different countries such as Negros generally have 5 to 7 inches in length, when un-excited and 8 to 10 inches , when excited. But remember one thing that during erected condition 4 inches length of penis is sufficient for sexual satisfaction by both as it will touch the "Cervix" of female organ. Additional length of penis will be adjusted automatically in vagina without making any pain to female. It is used as an enjoyment tool. It is also used as a passage for passing semen and urine.

2. **Corpus cavernosum (3 nos.)**: It is sponge-like region of erectile tissue. When male excited, blood get trapped inside the tissue and could not get out. Thus penis gets erected.

3. **Corpus spongiosum**: It is like a tube. Main purpose is to prevent urethra (urine) to enter in to penis passage, when penis is in erected condition.

4. **Foreskin of Glans**: It is skin, which covers the Glans. After intercourse several times this skin remains uncover permanently. Muslims cut the foreskin at boyhood itself and it is known as Circumcision.`.

5. **Glans**: It is known as "Head of Penis". It is most sensitive sex organ. Peculiarity in shape: It is round, conical and probe-like shape and top portion is having bigger diameter with a slot where as bottom portion is having smaller diameter. Thus it will smoothly penetrate inside vagina, but will not be able to come out of vagina easily due to bigger diameter with a slot during upward stroke of intercourse.

6. **Scrotum**: It is the loose pouch-like sac of skin that hangs behind the penis. It contains 2 nos. testicles, (also called testes), as well as many nerves and blood vessels. It has a protective function and acts as a climate control system . For normal sperm development, the testes must be at a temperature slightly cooler than the body temperature. Special muscles in the wall of the scrotum allow it to contract and relax,

moving the testicles closer to the body for **warmth and protection or farther away from the body to cool the temperature.**

7. **Testicle / Testes (2 nos.)**: They consist of extremely small tubes, which contain blood vessels. Main purpose is to produce semen, which will be discussed later on. Size of each Testicle: 1.5 inches in length and 1 inch in breath. Left side Testicle is having more weight than other one, thus left Testicle hangs more. The testes are responsible for making testosterone (the primary male sex hormone) and for generating sperm. Within the testes are coiled masses of tubes called seminiferous tubules. These tubules are responsible for producing the sperm cells through a process called spermatogenesis.

8. **Epididymis (2 nos.)**: It is a curved structure and a long, coiled tube that rests on the backside of each testicle. Here sperm is stored and get matured.

9. **Urinary bladder**: It is nothing but a reservoir / storage for urine.

10. **Prostate gland**: It is a walnut-sized gland, located between bladder and penis and in front of rectum. Urethra runs through the centre of Prostate from bladder to penis. Prostate gland secretes the fluid that

nourishes and protects sperm. The urethra, which carries the ejaculate to be expelled during orgasm, runs through the center of the prostate gland.

11. **Urethra**: It is a tube, which connects urinary bladder so that urine could come out of body. In males, it has the additional function of expelling (ejaculating) semen, when the man reaches orgasm. When the penis is erected during sexual excitement, the flow of urine is blocked from the urethra, allowing only semen to be ejaculated at orgasm.

(B) FEMALE SEX ORGANS:

Short description of female sex organs:

The main female sex organs are as follows:

External parts:

1. Vulva / Vagina (outer)
2. Anus

Internal parts:

1. Vagina
2. Labium majora
3. Labium minora
4. Hymen

5. Clitoris
6. Cervix
7. Uterus (Womb)
8. Fallopian Tubes (2 nos.)
9. Ovaries (2 nos.)

1. **Vagina**: It is like a cannel, having elastic walls and expands to accumulate a penis of any size so that female do not get pain for bigger penis. During intercourse it is most sensitive organ. It is used for 3 purposes such as for sex, birthing (baby comes out of this canal) and menstrual blood is released from the body through this canal.
    It is usually six to seven inches in length, and its walls are lined with mucus membrane.

2. **Labium majora**: Outer lips of vagina. It has pubic hair.

3. **Labium minora**: Inner lips of vagina. It is sensitive and expands , when sexually stimulated.

4. **Hymen**: It is a thin membrane that covers entire vagina entrance. Main purpose is to keep germs and dirt out of vagina. It may get torn out during sports or other heavy physical activities. Thus it is not the indication for virginity at-all as someone thinks so.

5. **Clitoris**: **It is Known as "ladies' penis"**. It is like a button & filled with blood. It is made of many nerves and most sensible sex part and expands like balloon, when stimulated even by touching by hand also.

6. **Cervix**: It is a narrow entry point between uterus and vaginal cannel. During erected condition 4 inches length of penis is sufficient for sexual satisfaction by both as it will touch this "Cervix".

7. **Uterus**: It is known as womb. It looks like an up-side down pear. Main purpose is to hold and feed a developing fetus ,ie, future baby. Inner layer of uterus is made of blood and known as 'Endometrium". During menses period these blood comes out through vagina.

8. **Fallopian Tubes (2 nos.)**: They are tubes, which Connect Uterus with Ovaries. Thus eggs travel from ovaries to uterus through these tubes.

9. **Ovaries (2 nos.)**: They are primary organs of the reproductive system. They are of size of almonds and sit on each side of uterus. They produce ova / egg cell (generally one in each menstrual cycle) and female sex hormones (,ie, Estrogen and Progesterone). Each egg is held in a capsule (ie, Follicle). A matured egg bursts from follicle and known as Ovulation.

10. **Anus**:It is mainly used for the passage for stools to come out of body. But a few person used it as sex organ. It is better not to use it as sex tool. Because that process may rapture the passage or lead to some diseases.

(C)INDIRECT SEX ORGAN: Breast (Female)

(a).General Description:

Breast is not only sex organ, but also acts as most useful organ to living being, specially human being for the following reasons:

1. For great pleasure during pre-love play and intercourse.
2. For feeding to new born, which proved as only and only safe and anti-diseases food for new born.
3. For making female more beautiful as well as attractive.

For maintaining the body beautiful and attractive, some female do not feed her new born child properly. Because feeding longer period may cause slackness of her breast and thus attraction towards her may reduce. It is true that breast milk and feeding will cause slackness of her breast. But breast feed is unavoidable for the shake of new born child. Only two things she should be cautious as follows:

1. Too much pressure / thrust should not be put on breast.
2. Pressing the breast to be done by upward movement, not downward movement.

Size of breast:

Size of breast depends the following factors:

1. Heredity
2. Environment
3. Place, where lives , geographical conditions, atmosphere.
4. Food habit etc. etc.

Breast Massage:

Method: Massage will be done by hand with any massage oil or simply coconut oil.

Process: Movement of hand will be clockwise and anti-clockwise alternatively.

Precaution:Thrust of force of hand must be UP-WARD, not downward.

Advantages:
1. It develops bigger size of breast, which makes more attractive.

2. It keeps breast nerves, tissues etc. more active and alive.

Notes:

1. Massage can be done by self. But it will be better, if the same is done by other.
2. All females, whether having big or small breast, must do breast massage at least periodically. It will prevent the BREAST CANCER, which is now-a-days a common disease in modern society.

(b).Medical Description:

Breasts generally refers to front of chest and medically known as "Mammary glands". These glands are milk producing structures, composed of mainly fat cells.

Breast tissue of both male and female consists of tubular structure, known as "Ducts".

Female Breast:

At puberty female's ovaries produce female hormone, ie, "Estrogen", which causes the ducts to grow and also milk glands, ie, "Lobules" to develop at end of ducts. Amount of fat and connective tissue in breast also increases as female reaches puberty. These lobules can produce milk, when they receive the appropriate hormonal stimulation. Breast ducts transfer milk from lobules out to nipples and then milk exits from nipples while sucking.

Male Breast:

Please note that here is the deference for male. Male hormones, ie, "Testosterone" suppress the growth of breast tissue and lobules. <u>This is the reason that male breast does not grow at puberty.</u>

CHAPTER III

Penis, Potency/Impotency, Fertility

For sexual intercourse purpose penis of male is the first and foremost tool, which has to take the leading roll on this field. Thus little details of penis is discussed in this chapter.

Function of penis:

The penis contains a number of very sensitive nerves. The penis is the male main organ for sexual intercourse as well as passing urine. It has mainly 3 parts as follows:

1. Root: It attaches to the wall of the abdomen and remains inside the body.

2. Body or Shaft: It is cylindrical in shape and consists of 3 internal chambers, made up of special and sponge-like erectile tissue. This tissue contains thousands of large spaces that get filled with blood, when male is sexually excited. As these large spaces get filled with blood , then body of penis becomes

rigid and erected, which allows the penis to penetrate in to vagina of female during sexual intercourse. The skin of the penis is loose and elastic to accommodate changes in penis size during erection. When the male reaches the orgasm (sexual climax), semen with sperm is expelled (ejaculated) through the end of the penis with a great force. When the penis is erected, the flow of urine is blocked from the urethra and allowing only semen to be ejaculated at orgasm.

3. Glans: It is cone-shaped end of the penis. The glans, which also is called the head of the penis, is covered with a loose layer of skin, called foreskin. (This skin is sometimes removed in a procedure called circumcision.) The opening of the urethra, the tube that transports semen and urine, is at the tip of the glans.

Erection of penis:

An erection means the stiffening and rising of the penis, which occurs during sexual arousal, though it can also happen in non-sexual situations. The primary physiological mechanism that brings about erection is the autonomic dilation of arteries supplying blood to the penis, which allows more blood to fill the three spongy erectile tissue chambers in the penis, causing it to lengthen and stiffen. The now-engorged erectile tissue presses against and constricts the veins that carry blood away from the penis. More blood enters than leaves the penis, until an equilibrium is reached where an equal volume of blood flows into the dilated arteries and out of the constricted veins. Then a constant erectile size is achieved at this equilibrium. Erection facilitates sexual intercourse though it is not essential for various other sexual activities.

Erection angle:

Although many erect penises point upwards (see above soft pictures), it is common and normal for the erect penis to point nearly vertically upwards or nearly vertically downwards or even horizontally straight forward, all depending on the tension of the suspensory ligament that holds it in position.

The following table shows how common various erection angles from vertically upwards are for a standing male. In the table, zero degrees is pointing straight up against the abdomen, 90 degrees is horizontal and pointing straight forward, while 180 degrees would be pointing straight down to the feet. An upward pointing angle is most common. Please note that male should not worry un-necessary about erection of penis properly or not.

Angle (°)	Percent
0–30	5
30–60	30
60–85	31
85–95	10
95–120	20
120–180	5

Ejaculation / Discharge:

Ejaculation / Discharge is the ejecting of semen from the penis, and is usually accompanied by orgasm. A series of muscular contractions delivers semen, containing male gametes, known as sperm cells or spermatozoa, from the penis. It is usually the result of sexual stimulation, which may include prostate stimulation. (Rarely, it is due to prostatic disease). Ejaculation may occur spontaneously during sleep (known as a nocturnal emission or wet dream). Anejaculation is the condition of being unable to ejaculate.

Ejaculation has two phases: *emission* and ejaculatory. The emission phase of the ejaculatory reflex is under control of the sympathetic nervous system, while the ejaculatory phase is under control of a spinal reflex. A refractory period succeeds the ejaculation, and sexual stimulation precedes it.

Penis Disorders:

1. Erectile dysfunction is the inability to develop and maintain an erection sufficiently firm for satisfactory sexual performance. Diabetes is a leading cause, as is natural aging. A variety of treatments exist, including drugs, such as *sildenafil citrate* (marketed as Viagra), which works by vasodilation.

2. Paraphimosis is an inability to move the foreskin forward, over the glans. It can result from fluid trapped in a foreskin left retracted, perhaps following a medical procedure, or accumulation of fluid in the foreskin because of friction during vigorous sexual activity.

3. In diabetes, peripheral neuropathy can cause tingling in the penile skin and possibly reduced or completely absent sensation. The reduced sensations can lead to injuries for either partner and their absence can make it impossible to have sexual pleasure through stimulation of the penis. Since the problems are caused by permanent nerve damage, preventive treatment through good control of the diabetes is the primary treatment. Some limited recovery may be possible through improved diabetes control.

4. In Peyronie's disease, anomalous scar tissue grows in the soft tissue of the penis, causing

curvature. Severe cases can benefit from surgical correction.

5. A Thrombosis can occur during periods of frequent and prolonged sexual activity, especially fellatio. It is usually harmless and get cured automatically after some rest.

Penis Circumcision:

It means complete removal of the foreskin from the penis. As per record 30% male in the world are circumcised, some ones shortly after birth and some ones at adolescence. Please be noted that it is good for health on hygienic ground. Reasons are as follows:

1. The skin of circumcised penis becomes "Regular skin" like skin of arm / leg. Thus no dust / germs can stick there and can be cleaned easily.

2. The inner lining of foreskin (which is removed during circumcision) has many of cells, where HIV disease likes to intact. Thus it can prevent the spread of HIV .

3. Since the skin of circumcised penis can be kept clean easily, I will also help to prevent other diseases of STD etc.4. As per W.H.O.

report, circumcised male gets comparatively less victim of STD.

Penis Massage:

Method: Massage by hand with any massage oil or simple coconut oil.

Process:
1. Movement of hand will be forward and rear alternatively.
2. Movement of hands will be like the procedure, by which cow is being milked manually by bare hands in some countries. Here movement of both hands will be simultaneously and one after other.
3. Massage may be done only on the Glans (Head of penis) by one hand. It will reduce the sensitiveness of penis faster.

Advantages:
1. It develops bigger size penis. If penis size is less than 4 inches, then it is necessary.
2. It keeps penis nerves, tissues etc. active and alive.
3. Regular penis massage reduces the sensitiveness of penis. Thus it will INDIRECTLY helps to increase the duration of sexual intercourse due to loss of sensitiveness of penis.

Note: Though penis massage develops bigger size of penis, but generally it is not required. Because normally penis size in erected condition is more than 5 inches, where as 4 inches length is sufficient for sexual satisfaction by both as it touches the "Cervix" of female organ.

Potency:

Potency is the ability to take part in intercourse. If not able to do intercourse, then it is called "impotency". It is often called "Erectile Dysfunctiont". It is applicable to male (generally age of 12 to death) only, because female is having a simple hole , known as "vagina", where male has to insert his penis and penis entry is only possible, if penis remains rigid and stiff.

See Sl. No. 2 of MALE SEX ORGANS. Corpus cavernosum (2 nos.) are sponge-like region of erectile tissue. When male get sexually excited, blood get trapped inside the tissue and could not come out. Thus penis get erected and enlarged.

Reasons for Impotency:

(A) Mentally depression due to some reasons.

(B) Blood not getting trapped inside the Corpus cavernosum. Thus penis is not get erected and enlarged. Since penis does not remains rigid and stiff, he can not insert his penis into vagina.

(C) Some other physical deficiencies.

Treatment for Impotency:

(A) If it is due to depression, he himself should check and control his mind.

(B) If still not successful, he should not hesitate to consult Doctor for the problem.

Please note that now-a-days male is using a drug sildenafil citrate for erection of penis for longer period or as a treatment for impotency. It is sold under the brand name Viagra. Primary drawback of Viagra is that it works about an hour after it is taken. More over it is harmful for diabetes, high blood pressure etc. Thus it is recommended to use it after consultation with Doctor only.

Fertility:

It is the ability to reproduce ,ie, to give birth of child (generally one, sometimes may be more). It is applicable to male (generally age of 12 to death) as well as to female too (generally age of 12 to 50). It is a joint action. If any one of them is having fertility deficiency, then reproduction is not at all possible.

Fertility is directly related to the following factors:

(A) Sperm of semen of male is capable. (specially head of sperm must be sharp and pointed so that it can pears through the hard casing of ova of female) .

(B) Ova must be healthy.

(C) Uterus (Womb) of female must be suitable for *fetus's growth.*

Please remember that impotency may create difficult in intercourse time, but still if that male having fertility on his sperm, he can take part in reproduction by inserting the sperm into vagina artificially.

CHAPTER IV

MENSTRUATION CYCLE / MENSES:

Menstruation is also called menstrual bleeding, menses, catamenia or a period. It is the periodic blood that flows as a discharge from the uterus, when female does not get pregnant. It is applicable to female (generally age of 12 to 50).

An average cycle is 28 days, but anywhere from 23 to 35 days is also to be treated as normal. One egg cell ,ie, ova from ovaries get matured for production of new born once in a month. If ova meets the able sperm, pregnancy occurred and then thereafter no menses.

If ova could not meet the able sperm, then menses started for the following reason:

Inner layer of uterus is made of blood and known as 'Endometrium". This layer grows thicker by discharge of one type of hormone (FSH). If no pregnancy is occurred, then this thick blood layer only comes out through vagina as menses.

Thus menses indicate that no pregnancy occurred.

It is better to avoid intercourse during menses period because this blood is not good for health and may cause itching. But if it not possible to avoid intercourse due to some reasons, then intercourse may be done with protection like using cap on penis. It is true that a few female (not all) may feel more sexual appeal during this period. Generally female lose an average of about 2 ounces (60 ml) of blood during normal menstruation. Sometimes it is observed that matured female missed her menses, but not at-all pregnant. It may happen due to over stress and mentally upset. If it is occurred for some other reason, Gynecologist is to be consulted without fail.

Irregular cycles or irregular periods is an abnormal variation in length of menstrual cycles. A matured female usually experiences cycle length variations of up to 8 days between the shortest and longest cycle lengths. Length variation between 8 and 20 days is considered as moderately irregular cycles. Length variation of 21 days or more is considered very irregular. Alternatively a single menstruation period may be defined as irregular if it is shorter than 21 days or longer than 36 days. However if they are regularly shorter than 21 days or longer than 36 (or 35) days, the condition would rather be termed polymenorrhea or oligomenorrhea respectively.

Precautions during menses:

1. Blood of menses is mixed with various chemicals, which is harmful to health. Thus female has to take an extra precaution to keep the vagina cleaned. So she should make practice to clean the vagina with soap-water after urination.

2. She should take care of food as there are chances of indigestion during this period.

3. She should avoid physical hard works, which will cause more bleeding discharge.

4. Homeopathic medicine, ie, <u>PALSATILA is widely used as a remedy of the following problems:</u>

   A. To reduce the stomach pain prior to start of menses, if occurs.

   B. To regularize the irregularity of menses, if occurs.

   C. To regularize the quantity of menses (more-less) , if occurs.

Menstruation Phases:

**Menstruation cycle can be divided into 5 Phases.
First 3** phases are related to the changes of lining
of uterus, where as final 2 phases are related
processes occurring in ovary as follows:

Phases	Start day	End day	Duration / Day
Menstruation/Menstrual phase	1	5	5
*Pro-liferative phase	5	13	9
Ovulation/Ovulatory phase	13	16	4
Luteal/Secretory phase	16	28	13
Ischemic phase	27	28	2

*Pro-liferative phase: It is called Pro-liferative,
because during this period one type of hormone
(FSH) is produced. This hormone causes the lining
of the uterus to grow in order to take care of future
new-born. If pregnancy does not occur, then this
lining of the uterus along with blood will come out as
menses.

Sufferings during menstruation cycle:

1. Painful cramping in abdomen, back or upper
   thighs is very common.

2. Severe uterine pain, known as 'Dysmenorrhea" is
   common among adolescent and younger female.

Note:

Pre-menstrual syndrome such as breast tenderness and irritability etc. are generally getting reduced day by day after starting of menstruation.

Pregnancy Phases:

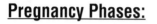

Line Diagram of Menstruation Circle :
(Considering a cycle of 28 days)

| 1 | 5 | 10 | 14-15 | 22 | 28 |

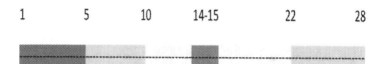

Now look at above Line Diagram considering a cycle of 28 days of a female.

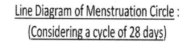 : Represents Menses period (Discharge of blood)

: Represents Save period (Chances of pregnancy is less)

---- : Represents Un-save period (Chances of pregnancy is more)

: Represents Ovulation period (Chances of pregnancy is maximum)

Menopause:

It is one of status of female, when menstruation cycle get stopped. Generally this status comes, when female attains 45 years or more. Though it is applicable to female only, but sometimes somebody say about Male Menopause, when penis of male not get erected due to over-age or some other reasons.

CHAPTER V

PRE-LOVE PLAY, INTERCOURSE (COITUS), ORGASM AND MASTURBATION

At first we must know the sex parts of male and female. Before proceeding further, we must have a fair knowledge on the following matters:

1. <u>Pre-love play</u>:

It is the activities, being done since sex appeal starts and continue up to entering the penis in to vagina. Pre-love play is a combine pair game, where both male and female must take part actively. But in practical field, it is observed that male takes more active part than female. Some females hesitate to take active part on it with a wrong concept that her partner may get wrong impression on her character. During love game, first of all, hugged themselves tightly for some times. Then sensitive parts of both are to be touched, pressed, kissed, sucked etc.

Sensitive parts are as follows (starting from minimum to maximum sensitive parts):

A. Fore head
B. Shoulder
C. Under arms
D. Abdomen
E. Thighs
F. Legs
G. Feet
H. Hip
I.   Breast / Breast nipples
J. Vagina of female
K. Clitoris of vagina
L. Testicles of male
M. Penis of male (mainly head)

It is to be noted that male must not touch the clitoris without pre-love play, otherwise female may feel uneasy / pain.

Duration of Pre-love play: No limit, but continue till liquid being getting discharged from penis and vagina.

2. Intercourse (Coitus):

Intercourse is nothing but a sexual union between a male and female involving insertion of the penis of male into the vagina of female. Intercourse means continuous movement of penis inward and outward inside the vagina without disconnecting them. During inward movement / stroke, foreskin of penis opens out from forehead and penis head rubes directly on the inner wall of vagina. Then it makes more sense of pleasure. During outward movement / stroke, foreskin of penis gets closed and come to previous location. In this way inward and outward stroke goes on till orgasm occurs.

There are other types of intercourse, where pair of a male and a female or of a male and male are involved. They are as follows:

(A) Oral Intercourse, where penis inserts into mouth. It is common in the world. But here cleanness of penis must be taken care of.

(B) Anus Intercourse, where penis inserts into anus. Though it is not common in many countries, but it has a wide use. It is not advisable at-all. It may cause the tear of the passage of anus. Even it may cause for some diseases also.

NOTES:

1. Please do not forget that both players (ie, male and female) have a common goal that is 100% satisfaction in the sex field (ie, sexual intercourse). To achieve it both MUST COOPERATE each other. Even if any one has any deficiency, other has to help / assist to overcome that deficiency. Otherwise both

will be <u>at lost</u> in the sex game and then it may lead to divorce at the end.

2. Details of intercourse with 60 postures and how to stimulate sex desire etc. will be mentioned in next chapter.

3. <u>Orgasm</u>:

Orgasm is the highest point of sexual excitement, characterized by strong feelings of pleasure and marked normally by ejaculation of semen by the male and by vaginal contractions by the female. It is also called climax.

It means <u>male enjoys orgasm (ie, pleasure of intercourse) by discharging semen, where as female enjoys it by vaginal contraction.</u>

By nature male gets excited within short period, but female gets excited after longer period.

Now look at the following Excitement Diagrams:

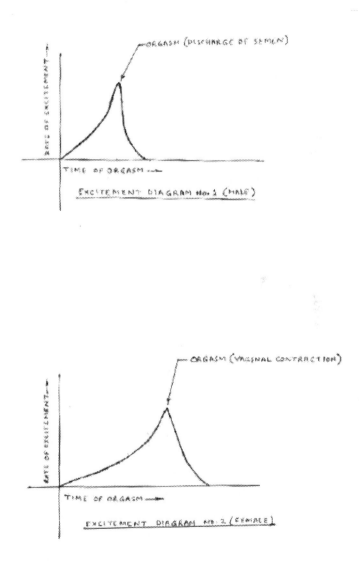

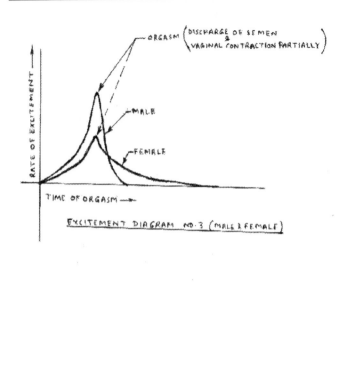

ORGASM (DISCHARGE OF SEMEN & VAGINAL CONTRACTION PARTIALLY)

MALE

FEMALE

RATE OF EXCITEMENT →

TIME OF ORGASM →

EXCITEMENT DIAGRAM NO. 3 (MALE & FEMALE)

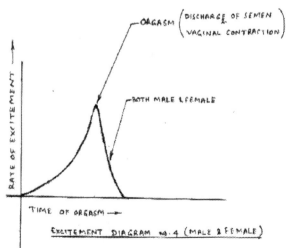

ORGASM (DISCHARGE OF SEMEN & VAGINAL CONTRACTION)

BOTH MALE & FEMALE

RATE OF EXCITEMENT →

TIME OF ORGASM →

EXCITEMENT DIAGRAM NO. 4 (MALE & FEMALE)

In Excitement Diagram No. I, time of orgasm for the same amount of excitement is less in case of male.

In Excitement Diagram No. 2, time of orgasm for the same amount of excitement is more in case of female.

In Excitement Diagram No. 3, if time of orgasm is maintained the same during intercourse, then male can reach the peak point of excitement, ie, orgasm in time, whereas female can not reach the peak point and has to walk off on half the way. Here male enjoys the sex, but female gets it partially.

Since it is a common and nature phenomena, now we should do something to overcome this deficiency. Thus we have to make sure that female gets orgasm faster and at the same time male gets it later. There are the following three remedies to overcome this deficiency:

1. Before starting of actual intercourse, pre-love play is to be continued for longer period so that excitement of female reaches near orgasm.

2. Before inserting the penis in to vagina, a little oil, preferable coconut oil, is to be put on the head of penis/glans. This oil will be utilized as lubrication. Thus it will reduce the friction between the penis and the inside wall of vagina. Once the friction is reduced, then excitement feeling also will be

reduced. Ultimately duration of intercourse time will be increased.

Note:

(A) During excitement female discharges various types of secretions. These secretions also act as lubrication. Since female gets excited at slower rate than male, thus additional oil on penis will help for faster lubrication.

(B) These secretions have a specialty of smelling, which makes the male attracted and sexually excited.

(C) If these secretions remain inside the vagina for longer period, they get spoiled and cause for itching.

Thus female must make habit to clean the inside of vagina periodically and at-least once in a day with soap-water.

3. During intercourse time, Just little before discharge of semen, male has to do two things:

(A) To divert his attention of mind to other matter so that his excitement gets reduced.

(B) To hold his breathing as much as possible.

It is not an easy job. It <u>requires some practice</u>; then only he will be able to control his discharge of semen as and when he wants.

<u>In</u> Excitement Diagram No. 4, these above remedy procedures are utilized. Thus both male and female excitement diagrams are on the same line. Here discharge of semen of male and vagina contraction of female are happened at the same time. Thus here both <u>male and female enjoy the sex</u> and left bed with smiling face.

5. <u>Masturbation</u>:

It is a very innocent means / medium for relaxing sexual tensions. It is an auto-eroticism. The person tries to derive sex pleasure by self-manipulations and does not need a partner of opposite sex. Off-course mutual masturbation among companions of same sex is fairly common. It is safe, natural and healthy. It should not be treated as unusual or abnormal. Even it is not harmful, if it is not excessive. It will be harmful, when it becomes habit or essential, without which other thing getting disturbed. As for example: If a person does not get sleep without masturbation, in this case it is harmful. <u>A child learns masturbation quite spontaneously and accidently, while pondling genitals (penis / vagina).</u>

(A) <u>Male masturbation</u>: Male masturbation is nothing but pressing and pushing the foreskin of penis forward and back continuously by own hand till orgasm takes place. It is not only common for male, but also each male must has experience of it. Now-a-days sex tools like dildo or vibrator for male are available in most of countries. Their uses are limited .

(B) <u>Female masturbation</u>: Female masturbation is all about having an orgasm without the help of male partner. It can involve clitoral stimulation or deeper penetration of own fingers or something else in vagina. It is not common among female. Some female may not have experience of masturbation in her whole life. Now-a-days sex tools like dildo or vibrator for female are also available in most of countries. But their uses are very much limited.

CHAPTER VI

DETAILS OF INTERCOURSE POSTURES

*How to stimulate the sex desire and keep sexual attraction alive towards Life partner throughout the life? This question is common for all married persons. Even this is the question, which inspires me to write this book.

Sex is nothing but one type of hungers for living creatures. We take food daily several times to fulfill our hunger. In addition matured persons feel hunger for sex also. Only difference is that this sex hunger is not several times. It is only once and that too not daily, periodically as per personal desire and at favorable environment. If environment is not suitable, then hunger for sex also will not be felt. Thus in bad status of mind, we are not in a position to do intercourse.

We get bored, if same type of foods are served again and again. Thus we try to prepare our foods in different ways every time for change of test on food, though food materials (like rice, chapatti, vegetables, mutton etc.) remain same.

Similarly we also get bored and exhausted to have sex with same life partner again and again. Thus like change of test on food, we also have to change the test on sex with same partner only by adopting different intercourse postures every time.

60 types Intercourse Postures:

Here 60 types Intercourse Postures are mentioned. Any advantage / disadvantage on that posture, advisable during pregnancy period, suitable for new couple, suitable for slag penis holder (whose penis gets erected in excitement, but does not hold stiffness for longer period due to some reason) etc. are mentioned in each and every posture. Some of them may look similar but little difference will be noticed, if looked carefully. Thus you must keep on changing the posture every time to stimulate the sex desire of yourself as well as your partner too. This is the way, by which you can keep the sexual attraction alive towards your partner throughout the live.

For saving your valuable time, it is prepared as a spoon-feed. Thus all these postures are categorized and sub-divisioned so that they can be viewed at a glance.

The great roll of worry-cum— mental tension on sex life-cum-marriage:

My dear all couples, please pay great attention on worry-cum—mental tension. In this ultra modern-cum—nuclear society, people (male or female or both) are remained or compelled to remain busy on their jobs / business for most of time of the day. Thus some additional problems are also accumulated on their lives. But they could not get adequate time to solve these problems. As a result, mental tension_arises. The mental tension will be doubled, when both (male and female) remain busy on their jobs for most of time. This mental tension definitely will make a great damage on their sex lives directly. Because during sex activities this mental tension directly / indirectly will re-appear in their mind automatically. Again as a result, their sex organs also will not perform satisfactory / properly. Then there will be "The END" on the half way of their sex play / sex activities. Thus both of them will not get 100% sex satisfaction. This sex dissatisfaction again will carry forward on next time and so keep on increasing. After sometime, this sex dissatisfaction itself will make so great problem , which may even lead to break the marriage also. <u>To overcome this great problem, both of you must be sure that both minds are completely free from all types of worry-cum—mental tension before starting of your sex play.</u>

Thus my sincere advise to my readers that you must make sure that no worry / tension should come in both minds during your sex play time and both of you must enjoy sex 100% with compete free minded.

Short Line Sketch: Not getting adequate time to solve their personal worry-cum—mental tension—Mental tension reappears automatically during sex play—Sex organs also will not perform satisfactory / properly—Couple will not get 100% sex satisfaction—This sex dissatisfaction again will carry forward and so keep on increasing—Later on it will make so great problem, which may even lead to break the marriage. Thus be <u>very cautious</u> on it.

Please note that it is easy to understand the postures, if they are in picture form. Since these short of pictures are not permitted, I will try to explain the postures only by language. Please excuse my in-ability, if I could not explain them properly.

There are mainly 4 categories of postures, such as:

- A. Laying down Postures:
  - a. Female bottom & male top
  - b. Male bottom & female top
- B. Sitting Postures
- C. Knee down Postures
- D. Standing Postures

Here some Main (Basic) Postures are mentioned. Then these Main Postures are elaborated with some modification / changes to make other postures. In this way total 60 postures are mentioned. Thus the difference between one posture to other posture may be very little. So you have to be very attentive to distinguish the difference from one posture to other one.

No. of <u>Main Postures (marked with *)</u>: 43

No. of Associated Postures: 17

Intercourse Postures with segregation at a glance:

Postures	Locations	Pages
1. Lay down:		
(a) Female bottom & male up:	Posture No. 1 to 21	60
(b) Male bottom & female up:	Posture No. 22 to 37	68
2. Sitting	Posture No. 38 to 45	73
3. Knee down	Posture No. 46 to 49	77
4. Standing	Posture No. 50 to 60	79

(A) Postures for new couple: Posture No. 1, 2, 3, 4, 5, 6, 31, 33, 35, 38, 39, 40, 45, 46, 47, 48, 49, 50, 51, 52, 53, 54, 55, 56.

(B) Postures for slag penis holder: Posture No. 1, 2, 3, 4, 5, 6, 31, 33, 35, 38, 39, 40, 45, 46, 47, 48, 49, 50, 51, 52, 53, 54, 55, 56.

(C) Postures for pregnancy period:

   (a) Safest at all stages: Posture No. 51, 52, 53.

   (b) No at advanced stage: Posture No. 1, 2, 3, 4, 5, 6, 12, 13, 14, 15, 16, 17, 31, 35, 36, 37, 38, 39, 40, 45, 46, 47, 48, 49, 50, 54, 55, 56.

   (c) No at all stages: Posture No. 7, 8, 9, 10, 11, 18, 19, 20, 21, 22, 23, 24, 25, 26, 27, 28, 29, 30, 32, 33, 34, 41, 42, 43, 44, 57, 58, 59, 60.

(A) Laying down Postures:

a. Female bottom & male top:

*Posture No. 1: Female is laying down at back with her legs folded & apart. Male also will lay down inside her legs with face to face, keeping his head up & balancing his body by keeping his hands on bed.

Remarks:
   A) Easy for new couple.
   B) Easy for slag penis holder (whose penis get stiff, but does not remain long time).
   C) Pregnant permitted, but not in advanced stage.

D) Deep penetration possible.

*Posture No. 2: As sl. no 1. Difference: Female will raise her hip little bit up & keep her balanced by holding male's shoulder by her two hands. Male also laying down inside her legs with head up & face to face.

Remarks:
   A) Easy for new couple.
   B) Easy for slag penis holder (whose penis get stiff, but does not remain long time).
   C) Pregnant permitted, but not in advanced stage.
   D) Deep penetration possible.

*Posture No. 3: As sl. no 1. Difference: Male will keep his head down. Both will embrace each other.

Remarks:
   A) Easy for new couple.
   B) Easy for slag penis holder (whose penis get stiff, but does not remain long time).
   C) Pregnant permitted, but not in advanced stage.
   D) Deep penetration possible.

*Posture No. 4: Female laying down at back with her legs up. Male will sit down in front of her hip with face to face & holding her legs up.

Remarks:
   A) Easy for new couple.
   B) Easy for slag penis holder (whose penis get stiff, but does not remain long time).
   C) Pregnant permitted, but not in advanced stage.
   D) Deep penetration possible.

*Posture No. 5: As sl. no 4. Difference: Female's legs will be held by herself.

Remarks:
   A) Easy for new couple.
   B) Easy for slag penis holder (whose penis get stiff, but does not remain long time).
   C) Pregnant permitted, but not in advanced stage.
   D) Deep penetration possible.

*Posture No. 6: As sl. no 4. Difference: Female's legs will be placed on either on both sides or on any one side of his shoulder.

Remarks:
   A) Easy for new couple.
   B) Easy for slag penis holder (whose penis get stiff, but does not remain long time).

    C) Pregnant permitted, but not in advanced stage.
    D) Deep penetration possible.

*Posture No. 7: As sl. no 4. Difference: Female's legs will be placed on <u>just below the male's shoulder</u> on both sides & then crossed / locked her on his back.

Remarks:
    A) Pregnant not permitted
    B) Deep penetration possible.

*Posture No. 8: As sl. no 4. Difference: Female's legs will be placed on <u>male's abdomen on both sides</u>. Male will be in doggy position.

Remarks:
    A) Pregnant not permitted.
    B) Deep penetration possible.

Posture No. 9: As sl. no 4. Difference: Female's legs will be placed on <u>male's abdomen on both sides & then crossed/locked her legs</u> on his back. Male will be in doggy position.

Remarks:
    A) Pregnant not permitted
    B) Deep penetration possible.

*Posture No. 10: Female laying down straight at back. Her legs may be <u>kept little apart, but not folded to facilitate the penis entry</u>. Male also <u>laying down on her top face to face.</u>

Remarks:
  A) Pregnant not permitted.
  B) Deep penetration not possible.

Posture No. 11: As sl. no. 10. Difference: Male also laying down on her top, but in <u>opposite face & towards her legs</u>. It means that male's legs will be in front of female's face & vice versa.

Remarks:
  A) Pregnant not permitted.
  B) Deep penetration not possible.

*Posture No. 12: Female <u>laying down & resting on one side only</u> (left or right side). Male also laying down, but at one side <u>face to face & in between her legs</u> & embracing each other.

Remarks:
  A) Pregnant permitted, but not in advanced stage.
  B) Deep penetration not possible.

Posture No. 13: As sl. no. 12. Difference: Male also laying down at one side <u>behind her hip</u> &will enter his penis from back.

Remarks:
   A) Pregnant permitted, but not in advanced stage.
   B) Deep penetration not possible.

Posture No. 14: As sl. no. 12. Difference: Male' legs will be in between her legs, but in <u>opposite to her face & towards her legs</u>. It means that male's legs will be in front of female's face & vice versa.

Remarks:
   A) Pregnant permitted, but not in advanced stage.
   B) Deep penetration not possible.

*Posture No. 15: As sl. no. 12. Difference: Both male & female will lay down on one side, <u>but crosswise like "X" (neither face to face nor opposite face)</u>.

Remarks:
   A) Pregnant permitted, but not in advanced stage.
   B) Deep penetration not possible.

*Posture No. 16: As sl. no. 12. Difference: Female laying down & resting on one side only(left or right side). But her <u>one leg is up & other one is down</u> on bed. Male is <u>sitting on her "down" leg & holding her "up" leg.</u>

Remarks:
- A) Pregnant permitted, but not in advanced stage.
- B) Deep penetration not possible.

*Posture No. 17: As sl. no. 12. Difference: Her <u>one leg is up & on male's shoulder</u> & other one is down on bed. Male is <u>sitting on her "down" leg.</u>

Remarks:
- A) Pregnant permitted, but not in advanced stage.
- B) Deep penetration not possible.

*Posture No. 18: Female laying down <u>at chest & keeping legs apart</u> & her <u>vagina will be put little up to facilitate the penis entry</u>. Male also laying down in <u>between her legs & keeping his face on her back</u>.

Remarks:
- A) Insert of penis into vagina will not be smooth.
- B) Pregnant not permitted.
- C) Deep penetration not possible.

Posture No. 19: As sl. no. 18. Difference: Male also laying down in between her legs but <u>keeping his face on her leg(s)</u>.

Remarks:
   A) Insert of penis into vagina will not be smooth.
   B) Pregnant not permitted.
   C) Deep penetration not possible.

*Posture No. 20: As sl. no 18. Difference: Male sitting on her hip.<u> But his one leg is in between her legs & his other leg will be outer side of her leg.</u>

Remarks:
   A) Insert of penis into vagina will not be smooth.
   B) Pregnant not permitted.
   C) Deep penetration not possible.

Posture No. 21: As sl. no. 18. Difference: Male sitting on her hip by <u>keeping his body bent backward & keeping his body balanced by his hands on bed.</u>

Remarks:
   A) Insert of penis into vagina will not be smooth.
   B) Pregnant not permitted.
   C) Deep penetration not possible.

b. Male bottom & female top:

*Posture No. 22: Male laying own at back with his both legs closed together. Female also laying down on him & face to face

Remarks:
   A) Insert of penis into vagina will not be smooth.
   B) Pregnant not permitted.
   C) Deep penetration not possible.

Posture No. 23: As sl. no. 22. Difference: Female laying down on him but in opposite face & towards her legs. It means that female's legs will be in front of male's face & vice versa.

Remarks:
   A) Insert of penis into vagina will not be smooth.
   B) Pregnant not permitted.
   C) Deep penetration not possible.

Posture No. 24: As sl. no. 22. Difference: Female also laying down at her back & on top of his back. Faces of both male & female will be in same side. Their positions is to be little adjusted during the entry of penis.

Remarks:
- A) Insert of penis will not be smooth.
- B) Pregnant not permitted.
- C) Deep penetration not possible.

Posture No. 25: As sl. no. 22. Difference: Female also laying down at her back & on top of his legs. Face of male will be opposite to that of female.

Remarks:
- A) Insert of penis into vagina will not be smooth.
- B) Pregnant not permitted.
- C) Deep penetration not possible.

*Posture No. 26: As sl. no. 22. Difference: Female sitting on him face to face.

Remarks:
- A) Insert of penis into vagina will not be smooth.
- B) Pregnant not permitted.
- C) Deep penetration not possible.

Posture No. 27: As sl. no. 22. Difference: Female sitting on him, but in opposite face.

Remarks:
- A) Insert of penis into vagina will not be smooth.
- B) Pregnant not permitted.
- C) Deep penetration not possible.

*Posture No. 28: As sl. no. 22. Difference: Female sitting on him, but <u>her face will be crosswise like "X"</u> (neither face to face nor opposite face).

Remarks:
    A) Insert of penis into vagina will not be smooth.
    B) Pregnant not permitted.
    C) Deep penetration not possible.

*Posture No. 29: Male laying down at back, but his both legs kept <u>folded & closed together</u>. Female sitting on him <u>face to face</u>.

Remarks:
    A) Insert of penis into vagina will not be smooth.
    B) Pregnant not permitted.
    C) Deep penetration not possible.

Posture No. 30: As sl. no 29. Difference: Female sitting on him, but in <u>opposite face</u>.

Remarks:
    A) Insert of penis into vagina will not be smooth.
    B) Pregnant not permitted.
    C) Deep penetration not possible.

*Posture No. 31: Male laying down at back, but his both legs kept <u>folded & apart</u> also. Female sitting in between his legs in <u>face to face</u>.

Remarks:
   A) Easy for new couple.
   B) Easy for slag penis holder (whose penis get stiff, but does not remain long time).
   C) Pregnant permitted, but not in advanced stage.
   D) Deep penetration possible.

Posture No. 32: As sl. no. 31. Difference: Female sitting in between his legs, but in <u>opposite face.</u>

Remarks:
   A) Pregnant not permitted.
   B) Deep penetration not possible.

*Posture No. 33: Male laying down at back, but his <u>both legs kept hanging & up</u>. Female <u>sitting in between his legs face to face & holding his hanging legs.</u>

Remarks:
   A) Easy for new couple.
   B) Easy for slag penis holder (whose penis get stiff, but does not remain long time).
   C) Pregnant permitted, but not in advanced stage.

D) Deep penetration possible

Posture No. 34: As sl. no. 33. Difference: Female sitting in between his legs , but in <u>opposite face & towards his legs & holding his hanging legs.</u>

Remarks:
A) Pregnant not permitted.
B) Deep penetration not possible.

*Posture No. 35: Male laying down at back, but <u>his both legs kept on either on both shoulders or on one side of shoulder of female</u> (left or right). Female sitting in between his legs <u>face to face</u>.

Remarks:
A) Easy for new couple.
B) Easy for slag penis holder (whose penis get stiff, but does not remain long time).
C) Pregnant permitted, but not in advanced stage.
D) Deep penetration possible.

*Posture No. 36: Male laying down & resting on one side (left or right). His <u>one leg is up & other one is down on bed. Female is sitting on his "down" leg & holding his "up" leg.</u>

Remarks:

    A) Pregnant permitted, but not in advanced stage.

    B) Deep penetration not possible.

Posture No. 37: As sl. no. 36. Difference: His <u>one leg is up & on her shoulder & other one is down on bed. Female is sitting on his "down" leg.</u>

Remarks:

    A) Pregnant permitted, but not in advanced stage.

    B) Deep penetration not possible.

B. <u>Sitting Postures</u>:

*Posture No. 38: Male is in sitting position with <u>his legs closed together & keeps his head backward. He balanced his body by keeping hands on bed</u>. His legs will be straight, not folded. Female <u>sits on his lap face to face </u>& embracing his neck.

Remarks:

    A) Easy for new couple.

    B) Easy for slag penis holder (whose penis get stiff, but does not remain long time).

    C) Pregnant permitted, but not in advanced stage.

    D) Deep penetration possible.

Posture No. 39: As sl. no. 38. Difference: Male is in sitting position, but his legs kept folded without any gap between his legs. Female sits on his lap face to face & embracing his neck.

Remarks:
   A) Easy for new couple.
   B) Easy for slag penis holder (whose penis get stiff, but does not remain long time).
   C) Pregnant permitted, but not in advanced stage.
   D) Deep penetration possible.

*Posture No. 40: As sl. no. 38. Difference: Male is in sitting position keeping his head backward & balanced by hand, but his legs kept folded loosely so that there will be a gap between his legs. Female will sit in between his legs. Both will embrace each other.

Remarks:
   A) Easy for new couple.
   B) Easy for slag penis holder (whose penis get stiff, but does not remain long time).
   C) Pregnant permitted, but not in advanced stage.
   D) Deep penetration possible.

*Posture No. 41: Male is in sitting position with <u>his legs closed together</u>. Female will <u>lay down on chest & on top of his legs in opposite face. She will keep her legs by the sides (left & right) of his abdomen.</u>

Remarks:
- A) Insert of penis into vagina will not be smooth.
- B) Pregnant not permitted.
- C) Deep penetration not possible.

Posture No. 42: As sl. no. 41. Difference: Male is in <u>normal sitting position</u>, but <u>his legs kept apart</u>. Female will <u>lay down on chest but in between this gap of his legs in opposite face</u>. She will keep her legs by the sides (left & right) of his abdomen.

Remarks: As above.

- A) Insert of penis into vagina will not be smooth.
- B) Pregnant not permitted.
- C) Deep penetration not possible.

*Posture No. 43: Male will sit on a tool, which has <u>no back rest</u>. Female will sit on his lap <u>face to face</u> embracing each other to keep their bodies balanced.

Remarks:
- A) Pregnant not permitted.
- B) Deep penetration not possible.

*Posture No. 44: As sl. no 43. Difference: Female will sit on his lap but <u>in opposite face</u>. Thus male will hold her body to keep her body balanced.

Remarks:
   A) Pregnant not permitted.
   B) Deep penetration not possible.

*Posture No. 45: Male will sit on bed keeping <u>his legs folded with a gap</u>. Female will sit in between this gap of his legs <u>face to face</u>. Both will embrace each other to keep their bodies balanced.

Remarks:
   A) Easy for new couple.
   B) Easy for slag penis holder (whose penis get stiff, but does not remain long time).
   C) Pregnant permitted, but not in advanced stage.
   D) Deep penetration possible.

C. Knee down Postures:

*Posture No. 46: Doggy position. Female will <u>rest on her legs & hands & parallel to bed</u>. Male will insert <u>penis to vagina from her back.</u>

Remarks:
- A) Easy for new couple.
- B) Easy for slag penis holder (whose penis get stiff, but does not remain long time).
- C) Pregnant permitted, but not in advanced stage.
- D) Deep penetration possible.

*Posture No. 47: Doggy position. Difference: Female will be <u>resting on her folded hands on bed. Her head also will be resting on bed so that her hip will be projected upward</u>, which will facilitate easy penis penetration. It means that <u>female's body will be at an angle</u>, resting one end on folded hands & heads, but other end on folded legs.

Remarks:
- A) Easy for new couple.
- B) Easy for slag penis holder (whose penis get stiff, but does not remain long time).
- C) Pregnant permitted, but not in advanced stage.
- D) Deep penetration possible.

*Posture No. 48: <u>3 or 4 pillows</u> are to be kept on bed. Female will rest on these beds on her chest. Male will be resting on her back.

Remarks:
   A) Easy for new couple.
   B) Easy for slag penis holder (whose penis get stiff, but does not remain long time).
   C) Pregnant permitted, but not in advanced stage.
   D) Deep penetration possible.

*Posture No. 49: Here place is <u>stair case</u>. Female will rest on the higher & broader stair case on her chest. Male will be resting on her back.

Remarks:
   A) Easy for new couple.
   B) Easy for slag penis holder (whose penis get stiff, but does not remain long time).
   C) Pregnant permitted, but not in advanced stage.
   D) Deep penetration possible.

D. Standing Postures:

*Posture No. 50: Male standing in front of bed, whose height should be <u>little below the penis height</u>. Female will be laying down on bed at her back & her legs will be <u>hold by male in CROSSED position</u>.

Remarks:
    A) Additional advantage for loose vaginal hole, which may occur due to medical surgery or overage or excessive use (prostitute). Because CROSSED legs make the vaginal hole smaller diameter & tightfitting.
    B) Additional advantage for slag penis holder too. Because it will make tight fitting.
    C) Easy for new couple.
    D) Pregnant permitted, but not in advanced stage.
    E) Deep penetration possible

*Posture No. 51: As sl. no. 50. Difference: Her legs will be <u>hold by male in OPENED position</u>.

Remarks:
    A) Easy for new couple.
    B) Easy for slag penis holder.
    C) Pregnant permitted in all stages & the easy as well as safest process.
    D) Deep penetration possible

*Posture No. 52: As sl. no. 50. Difference: Her legs will be kept <u>folded at the edge of the bed</u>.

Remarks:
- A) Easy for new couple.
- B) Easy for slag penis holder.
- C) Pregnant permitted in all stages & the easy as well as safest process.
- D) Deep penetration possible

*Posture No. 53: As sl. no 50. Difference: Her legs will be kept <u>on both sides of male's abdomen & then crossed/locked legs at his back.</u>

Remarks:
- A) Easy for new couple.
- B) Easy for slag penis holder.
- C) Pregnant permitted in all stages & the easy as well as safest process.
- D) Deep penetration possible

*Posture No. 54: As sl. no. 50. Difference: Her legs will be kept on <u>male' shoulder either on both shoulder or on one side shoulder.</u>

Remarks:
- A) Easy for new couple.
- B) Easy for slag penis holder.
- C) Pregnant permitted, but not in advanced stage.

D) Deep penetration possible

*Posture No. 55: Female will be standing & bend her body up to 90 degree keeping her legs apart & then keep <u>balanced her body by resting on a suitable height tool / chair.</u> Male will be at her back.

Remarks:
- A) Easy for new couple.
- B) Easy for slag penis holder.
- C) Pregnant permitted, but not in advanced stage.
- D) Deep penetration possible

*Posture No. 56: Female will be standing & bend her body up to 90 degree keeping her legs apart. Here her body will be <u>balanced by holding her hip by male.</u> Male will be at her back.

Remarks:
- A) Easy for new couple.
- B) Easy for slag penis holder (whose penis get stiff, but does not remain long time).
- C) Pregnant permitted, but not in advanced stage.
- D) Deep penetration possible

*Posture No. 57: Both male & female will be <u>standing & face to face</u>. Female has to bend backward little during entry of penis.

Remarks:
    A) Insert of penis into vagina will not be smooth.
    B) Pregnant not permitted.
    C) Deep penetration not possible.

*Posture No. 58: Both male & female will be standing, but male will be at her back. Female has to bend forward little during entry of penis.

Remarks:
    A) Insert of penis into vagina will not be smooth.
    B) Pregnant not permitted.
    C) Deep penetration not possible.

*Posture No. 59: Both male & female will be standing, but Female will stand on one leg. Her <u>other leg will be held by male by one hand</u> & by his other hand, he will held her hip to keep her body balanced.

Remarks:
    A) Insert of penis into vagina will not be smooth.
    B) Pregnant not permitted.
    C) Deep penetration not possible

Posture No. 60: Both male & female will be standing, but Female will stand on one leg. Her <u>other leg will be put on male's shoulder</u> & then male can hold her hip to keep her body balanced. (Female should have good height).

Remarks:
- A) Insert of penis into vagina will not be smooth.
- B) Pregnant not permitted.
- C) Deep penetration not possible.

CHAPTER VII

Pregnancy, Child birth and Status of New-born child

(A) <u>Pregnancy</u>

Pregnancy is the fertilization and development of one or more offspring, known as an "Embryo"or "Fetus"in a woman's uterus. In a pregnancy, there can be multiple gestations, as in the case of twins or more. Childbirth usually occurs about 38 weeks after conception in women (who have a menstrual cycle length of 4 weeks). This is approximately 40 weeks from the start of the last normal menstrual period. Conception can be achieved through sexual intercourse or assisted reproductive technology. An Embryo is the developing offspring during the first 8 weeks following conception and subsequently the term Fetus is used until birth. In medical or legal definitions, human pregnancy is somewhat arbitrarily divided into three trimester periods, as a means to simplify reference to the different stages of prenatal development. The first trimester carries the highest risk of miscarriage (natural death of embryo or fetus). During the second trimester, the development of the fetus can be more easily monitored and diagnosed. The beginning of the third trimester often approximates the point of viability or the ability of the fetus to survive, with or without medical help outside of the uterus

Although pregnancy begins with implantation, the process leading to pregnancy occurs earlier as the result of the female gamete or "Oocyte", merging with the male gamete or "Spermatozoon". In medical terms, this process is referred to as "Fertilization", but in lay terms and more commonly known as "Conception." After the point of fertilization, the fused product of the female and male gamete is referred to as a "Zygote"or fertilized egg. The fusion of male and female gametes usually occurs following the act of sexual intercourse, resulting in *spontaneous pregnancy*. However the advent of assisted reproductive technology such as artificial insemination and in vitro fertilisation have made achieving pregnancy possible without engaging in sexual intercourse. This approach may be undertaken as a voluntary choice or due to infertility.

The process of fertilization occurs in several steps and the interruption of any of them can lead to failure. Through fertilization the egg is activated to begin its developmental process and the haploid nuclei of the two gametes come together to form the genome of a new diploid organism. The sperm of male and the egg cell, which has been released from one of the female's two ovaries, unite in one of the two fallopian tubes. The fertilized egg, known as a Zygote, then moves toward the uterus. This journey may take up to a week to complete. Cell division begins approximately 24 to 36 hours after the male and female cells unite. Cell division continues at a rapid rate and the cells then develop into what is known as a Blastocyst. The blastocyst is made up of three layers: the ectoderm (which will become the skin and nervous system), the endoderm (which will become the digestive and respiratory systems) and the mesoderm (which will become the muscle and skeletal systems). Finally the blastocyst arrives at the uterus and attaches to the uterine wall. This process is known as Implantation.

The mass of cells, now known as an embryo, begins the embryonic stage, which continues until cell differentiation is almost complete at eight weeks. Then the embryo enters the final stage. This stage is known as a Fetus. The early body systems and structures that were established in the embryonic stage continue to develop. Sex organs begin to appear during the third month of gestation. The fetus continues to grow in both weight and length, although the majority of the physical growth occurs in the last weeks of pregnancy.

(B) <u>Child birth</u>:

Childbirth is the process whereby an infant is born. A sexually matured female is considered to be in labour when she begins experiencing regular uterine contractions, accompanied by changes of her cervix primarily effacement and dilation. While childbirth is widely experienced as painful, some female do report painless labours, while others find that concentrating on the birth helps to quicken labour and lessen the sensations. Most births are successful vaginal births but sometimes complications arise and a female may undergo a cesarean operation.

During the time immediately after birth, both the mother and the baby are hormonally cued to bond, the mother through the release of oxytocin, a hormone also released during breastfeeding. Studies show that skin-to-skin contact between a mother and her newborn immediately after birth is beneficial for both the mother and baby. A review done by the World Health Organization found that skin-to-skin contact between mothers and babies after birth reduces crying, improves mother-infant interaction, and helps mothers to breastfeed successfully. They recommend that neonates be allowed to bond with the mother during their first two hours after birth, the period that they tend to be more alert than in the following hours of early life.

Postnatal period:

The postnatal period begins immediately after the birth of a child and then extends for about six weeks. During this period, the mother's body begins the return to pre-pregnancy conditions that includes changes in hormone levels and uterus size.

Diagnosis:

The beginning of pregnancy may be detected either based on symptoms by the pregnant woman herself, or by using medical tests with or without the assistance of a medical professional.

Symptoms:

Most pregnant women experience a number of symptoms, which can signify pregnancy. The symptoms can include nausea and vomiting, excessive tiredness and fatigue, cravings for certain foods that are not normally sought out, and frequent urination particularly during the night.

Tests:

Pregnancy detection can be accomplished using one or more various tests, which detect hormones generated by the newly formed placenta. Blood and urine tests can detect pregnancy 12 days after implantation. Blood pregnancy tests are more sensitive than urine test.

First Trimester (Beginning to 12 weeks):

Traditionally medical professionals have measured pregnancy from a number of convenient points, including the day of last menstruation, ovulation, fertilization, implantation and chemical detection. Most pregnant women do not have any specific signs or symptoms of implantation, although it is not uncommon to experience minimal bleeding.

Morning sickness occurs in about seventy percent of all pregnant women, and typically improves after the first trimester. Although described as "morning sickness", female can experience this nausea during afternoon, evening, and throughout the entire day.

Shortly after conception, the nipples and areolas begin to darken due to a temporary increase in hormones. This process continues throughout the pregnancy.

The first 12 weeks of pregnancy are considered to make up the first trimester. The first 2 weeks from the first trimester are calculated as the first 2 weeks of pregnancy even though the pregnancy does not actually exist. These 2 weeks are the 2 weeks before conception and include the female's last period.

The 3rd. week is the week, in which fertilization occurs and the 4th week is the period, when implantation takes place. In the 4th week, the fecundated egg reaches the uterus and burrows into its wall which provides it with the nutrients it needs. At this point, the zygote becomes a blastocyst and the placenta starts to form. Moreover, most of the pregnancy tests may detect a pregnancy beginning with this week.

The 5th week marks the start of the embryonic period. This is when the embryo's brain, spinal cord, heart and other organs begin to form. At this point the embryo is made up of three layers, of which the top one (called the Ectoderm) will give rise to the embryo's outermost layer of skin, central and peripheral nervous systems, eyes, inner ear, and many connective tissues. The heart and the beginning of the circulatory system as well as the bones, muscles and kidneys are made up from the mesoderm (the middle layer). The inner layer of the embryo will serve as the starting point for the development of the lungs, intestine and bladder. This layer is referred to as the endoderm. An embryo at 5 weeks is normally between $\frac{1}{16}$ and $\frac{1}{8}$ inch (1.6 and 3.2 mm) in length.

In the 6th week, the embryo will be developing basic facial features and its arms and legs start to grow. At this point, the embryo is usually no longer than $\frac{1}{6}$ to $\frac{1}{4}$ inch (4.2 to 6.3 mm). In the following week, the brain, face and arms and legs quickly develop. In the 8th week, the embryo starts moving and in the next 3 weeks, the embryo's toes, neck and genitals develop as well. According to the American Pregnancy Association, by the end of the first trimester, the fetus will be about 3 inches (76 mm) long and will weigh approximately 1 ounce (28 g). Once pregnancy moves into the second trimester, all the risks of miscarriage and birth defects occurring drop drastically. Progesterone has noticeable effects on respiratory physiology, increasing minute ventilation by 40% in the first trimester.

Second Trimester (13 to 28 weeks):

By the end of the second trimester, the expanding uterus has created a visible "baby bump". Although the breasts have been developing internally since the beginning of the pregnancy. Most of the visible changes appear after this point.

Weeks 13 to 28 of the pregnancy are called the second trimester. Most female feel more energized in this period and begin to put on weight as the symptoms of morning sickness subside and eventually fade away.

The uterus, the muscular organ that holds the developing fetus, can expand up to 20 times its normal size during pregnancy.

Although the fetus begins to move and takes a recognizable human shape during the first trimester, it is not until the second trimester that movement of the fetus, often referred to as "Quickening", can be felt. This typically happens in the fourth month, more specifically in the 20th to 21st week or by the 19th week, if the female has been pregnant before. However it is not uncommon for some female not to feel the fetus movement until much later. The placenta fully functions at this time and the fetus makes insulin and urinates. The reproductive organs distinguish the fetus as male or female.

During the second trimester female should wear maternity clothes (loose clothes).

Third Trimester (29 weeks to Delivery):

Final weight gain takes place, which is the most weight gain throughout the pregnancy. The fetus will be growing the most rapidly during this stage, gaining up to 28 g per day. The female's belly will transform in shape as the belly drops due to the fetus turning in a downward position ready for birth. During the second trimester, the female's belly would have been very upright, whereas in the third trimester it will drop down quite low, and the female will be able to lift her belly up and down. The fetus begins to move regularly and is felt by the woman. Fetal movement can become quite strong and be disruptive to the female. The female's navel will sometimes become convex, "popping" out, due to her expanding abdomen. This period of her pregnancy can be uncomfortable, causing symptoms like weak bladder control and backache. Movement of the fetus becomes stronger and more frequent and via improved brain, eye and muscle function the fetus is prepared for *ex utero* viability. The female can feel the fetus "rolling" and it may cause pain or discomfort when it is near the female 's ribs and spine.

There is *head engagement* in the third trimester. The fetal head descends into the pelvic cavity so that only a small part (or none) of it can be felt abdominally. The perenium and cervix are further flattened and the head may be felt vaginally. Head engagement is known colloquially as the *baby drop*, and in natural medicine as the *lightening* because of the release of pressure on the upper abdomen and renewed ease in breathing. However it severely reduces bladder capacity, increases pressure on the pelvic floor and the rectum and the mother may experience the perpetual sensation that the fetus will "fall out" at any moment. It is also during the third trimester that maternal activity and sleep positions may affect fetal development due to restricted blood flow. For instance, the enlarged uterus may impede blood flow by compressing the lower pressured vena cava with the left lateral laying positions appearing to providing better oxygenation to the infant.

It is during this time that a baby born prematurely may survive. The use of modern medical intensive care technology has greatly increased the probability of premature babies surviving, and has pushed back the boundary of viability to much earlier dates than would be possible without assistance. In spite of these developments premature birth remains a major threat to the fetus and may result in ill health in later life, even if the baby survives.

Prenatal ultrasound imaging:

Prenatal development is divided into two primary biological stages. The first is the embryonic stage, which lasts for about two months. At this point the fetal stage begins. At the beginning of the fetal stage, the risk of miscarriage decreases sharply and all major structures including the head, brain, hands, feet and other organs are present, and they continue to grow and develop. When the fetal stage commences, a fetus is typically about 30 mm (1.2 inches) in length and the heart can be seen beating via ultrasound. The fetus can be seen making various involuntary motions at this stage.

Electrical brain activity is first detected between the 5th and 6th week of gestation, though this is still considered primitive neural activity rather than the beginning of conscious thought something that develops much later in fetation. Synapses begin forming at 17 weeks, and at about week 28 begin to multiply at a rapid pace which continues until 3 to 4 months after birth.

One way to observe prenatal development is via ultrasound images. Modern 3D ultrasound images provide greater detail for prenatal diagnosis than the older 2D ultrasound technology. While 3D is popular with parents desiring a prenatal photograph as a keepsake, both 2D and 3D are discouraged by the FDA for non-medical use.

Physiological changes:

During pregnancy the woman undergoes many physiological changes, which are entirely normal including cardiovascular, hematologic, metabolic, renal and respiratory changes that become very important in the event of complications. The body must change its physiological and homeostatic mechanisms in pregnancy to ensure the fetus is provided for. Increases in blood sugar, breathing and cardiac output are all required. Levels of progesterone and oestrogens rise continually throughout pregnancy, suppressing the hypothalamic axis and subsequently the menstrual cycle.

Similarly shape of breast changes during pregnancy. Its shape will keep on increasing at later stages accordingly.

Nutrition:

A balanced nutritious diet is an important aspect of a healthy pregnancy. Eating a healthy diet, balancing carbohydrates, fat and proteins, and eating a variety of fruits and vegetables usually ensures good nutrition.

Sexual activity:

Most women can continue to engage in sexual activity throughout pregnancy. Most research suggests that during pregnancy both sexual desire and frequency of sexual relations decrease. In context of this overall decrease in desire, some studies indicate a second-trimester increase, preceding a decrease during the third trimester. Sex during pregnancy is a low-risk behavior except when the healthcare provider advises that sexual intercourse be avoided for particular medical reasons. Otherwise for a healthy pregnant female, who is not ill or weak, can freely enjoy sex during pregnancy. It is enough to apply the common sense rule that both partners avoid putting pressure on the uterus or a partner's full weight on a pregnant.

As a safety measure, follow the intercourse postures, mentioned in the Chapter VI (Page:31): Details of Intercourse with 60 Postures.

(C). <u>Status of New-born child</u>:

Status of New-born child mainly depends on two factors:

    (a) Heredity
    (b) Environment

<u>(a) Heredit</u>y: New-born child inherits two sets of Gens (one from father and another from mother). The characteristics of the child depend on the combination/ result of these two gens. As for example: If the child inherits brown eyes from father and mother, his eyes will be brown. If the child inherits brown eyes from father and blue eyes from mother, his eyes will be brown, because brown color always dominates the blue. Again there is a different example: A child may get blue eyes , though his father and mother having brown eyes. Because his parents have genes for brown and blue also, though their eyes are brown. Thus the child gets these blue genes from parents. In this matter grandparent's genes also affect indirectly.

(b) Environment: Environment is a field/place, which provide multiple sources of stimulation to encourage the development of physical, mental, cognitive, emotional, and social skills to the child.

Note: Thus future of child is directly depends on these two factors:

(a) Heredity
(b) Environment

Comparison between them: Heredity is like Seed and Environment is like Soil of field. We know that if both seed and soil are good, we get bumper production. If one of them is not good, then production will be comparatively less. Here also if new-born child's heredity and environment are good, then child is expected (only) with prosperous future. But it does not mean that for prosperity of a child only good heredity and environment are required. It is being proved several times that a child made prosperous future, though child does not has good heredity or environment or both.

CHAPTER VIII

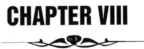

COMMON SEX RELATED PROBLEMS OF MALE AND FEMALE

Most of the so called sex diseases are psychological problems and are not the actual diseases. Most of these sex problems can be solved by sex counseling and need not any medicinal treatment. Even then some of these sex problems, which are prevailing since a long time effecting one's confidence and making him depressed may need medicine. Most of the anti-depressant medicines in modern system effect the sexual derive negatively so the best to overcome these type of problems are the Ayurvedic medicine, which increase sexual derive as well as improve confidence and are antidepressant also. Another group of medicines is <u>Homeopathic medicine, which is the best for persons with low confidence.</u>

Some of the actual sex diseases are the Sexually Transmitted Diseases (S.T.D.) and their complications even after the treatment with modern medicines like painful erections, premature ejaculation, atrophy of sex organism in male; vaginal dryness , dysparunia like painful intercourse and loss of orgasm in female; need Ayurvedic/Homeopathic treatment.

There is another group of sex diseases, which deal with sex organ anomalies like Phymosis etc. in male and like imperforated hymen etc. in female, which need surgical intervention. It is better to know about sex problems of male and female partners both, then only both the partners can get satisfied to-gether.

(A) Male sex problems /diseases:

1. Impotency: No or weak erection of penis without hardness even after strong stimulation by the female partner is called as "Impotency". The penis is unable to penetrate the vagina because of inefficient hardness of penis. Sometimes impotency may primarily be due to hormonal imbalance or may be temporary even after normal performance or due to psychological factor. In hormonal imbalance modern hormonal therapy is beneficial otherwise most of the cases may solved by counseling and or may need Ayurvedic/Homeopathic medicine.

    Please note that now-a-days male is using a drug sildenafil citrate, sold under the brand name Viagra. Primary drawback of Viagra is that it works about an hour after it is taken. More over it is harmful for diabetes, high blood pressure etc. <u>Thus it is recommended to use it after consultation with Doctor only.</u>

2. **Premature ejaculation (Discharge):** Normal time of actual penetrative sexual intercourse is 2 to 10 minutes. Ejaculation before 2 minutes or in other words before the satisfaction of partner is called as "Premature ejaculation". Premature ejaculation may be so early that it may be even before penetration or even without erection. Problem can be solved by counseling, if the time of ejaculation is more than 2 minutes as there may be female factors also as well as sex posture playing the important factor for sexual satisfaction of both the partners, while others may need Ayurvedic/Homeopathic medicine.

   To avoid **Premature ejaculation** a new technique is mentioned in the <u>CHAPTER I (Page:1): General knowledge on sex matters</u>, if there is no physical deficiency. Try to follow them.

3. **No orgasm:** No satisfaction after sexual intercourse due to no ejaculation of semen or very small Quantity of ejaculate otherwise normal erection and hardness. Needs medicine and best medicine in this case is Ayurvedic medicine.

4. **Blood stained ejaculate/semen:** This is the more aggravated form of the small quantity or no semen after sexual intercourse and needs Ayurvedic treatment but if the semen is blood

stained with large quantity of semen it may be due to some infection, which needs Allopathic medicine.

5. **Painful erection**: It is also due to small quantity of semen and needs Ayurvedic medicine, which is very good for production of semen.

6. **No interest in sexual indulgence**: Needs counseling or Ayurvedic / Homeopathic medicine or hormonal therapy .

7. **Phymosis**: Phymosis ie small opening of fore skin of penis due to which stimulations are weak. It can cause hindrance in erections. Needs surgical intervention.

8. **Long foreskin of penis**: Causes similar problem as Phymosis. Also needs surgical intervention.

9. **High attached and thick frenulum**: Frenulum is a fold of mucous membrane which attaches lower part of glans penis to the lower skin of shaft of penis.

Sometimes it is thick and attached high up to urethra which causes hindrance in erection and hardness ultimately causing curvature of shaft with convexity upward and concavity facing downward and also glans penis pointing downward even in erect position. This causes difficulty in penetration. Surgical intervention necessary. It is wise for the parents to see for the problem of Phymosis, long foreskin and high attached and thick frenulum in childhood and get that operated in time to avoid abnormal development of Penis.

10. **Small sized penis:** Normal size of penis during erection is about 5 inches to 9 inches, but with 4 inches size is enough to satisfy female, because normal size of vagina is 4 inches with at 3 inches Cervix length so the penis touches cervix easily to satisfy female. Moreover satisfaction of the woman depends more upon hardness, duration and the posture being used at the time of intercourse. Penis less than 4 inches needs treatment preferably Ayurvedic medicine. Massage on penis with any massage oil or simple coconut oil also helps to develop. See CHAPTER III (Page:35): Penis, Potency / Impotency, Fertility.

11. **Prostatorhoea:** Prostate secretion, a thick jelly like discharge at the time of passing stool and or urine. It can be treated Ayurvedically/ Homeopathically with very good results.

12. **Atrophy of sex organs:** Sex organs start shrinking after attaining the normal size which may be due to some disease or injury to the organs. Needs Ayurvdic/Homeopathic medicine.

(B) <u>Female sex problems/diseases</u>:

Females being the passive partner in sexual intercourse have very few sexual problems on their part. But <u>most of the sex problem of male arises from the improper behavior or non-cooperation of female during sexual intercourse</u>, which depend upon the sex problem female has at her own. So it is very important on the part of female also to get her problem solved and cooperate voluntarily and happily during sexual intercourse to have the best performances of her partner.

Common female sex problems are as follows:

1. **<u>Dysparunia:</u>** It is the pain during sexual intercourse. Thus disturbing attention at the time of intercourse, which affects orgasm and ultimately loss of sexual interest in female and also in male. Needs counseling and medicinal treatment, if necessary.

2. **<u>No interest in sexual indulgence</u>:** Needs counseling or Ayurvedic/Homeopathic medicine or hormonal therapy.

3. **<u>Vaginal inflamation and ulceration after every sexual intercourse</u>:** Requires counseling and medicinal treatment.

4. **<u>Vaginal itching</u>:** Requires medical advice for any infection.

5. **Imperforated hymen or semeperforated thick hymen:** It will cause pain. Thus avoiding penetration of penis during sexual intercourse. Needs surgical intervention.

6. **Small sized vagina unable to accommodate penis:** Only counseling can solve the problem in some cases, while others may need vaginal dilation or surgical intervention. It is very rare case.

7. **Atrophic or undeveloped sex organs:** May be hormonal problem. Needs hormonal investigations. Ayurvedic/Homeopathy can solve the problem in few cases.

8. **Gushing of fluid during sexual intercourse:** Needs medicinal treatment.

9. **Other genital infections causing Leukorhoea etc.:** It can alter sexual behavior and should be treated accordingly.

10. **Physical weakness after sexual intercourse:** Needs counseling and medicinal treatment in few cases.

Chapter IX

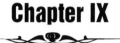

SEXUAL DISEASES

Sexually transmitted diseases (STDs) are caused by infections that are passed from one person to another during sexual contact. These infections often do not cause any symptoms. Medically infections are only called diseases when they cause symptoms.

There are many kinds of sexually transmitted diseases with two categories:

(A) **Viral Sexually Transmitted Diseases**:
1. HIV/AIDS
2. Genital Herpes
3. HPV and Genital Warts
4. Hepatitis

(B) **Bacterial Sexually Transmitted Diseases**:
1. Syphilis
2. Gonorrhea
3. Chancroid
4. Chlamydia
5. PID
6. Trichomoniasis

Among above diseases HIV/AIDS, Syphilis and
Gonorrhea are most common sexual diseases,
observed in India. Specially HIV/AIDS are spreading
here like a fire. Thus in this chapter HIV/AIDS are
discussed in little details.

Please make sure that whenever you have a
little suspect of attracting with STD, without fail
immediately consult with a V.D. Specialist and strictly
follow Doctor's instructions.

1. <u>HIV/AIDS</u>:

Human Immunodeficiency Virus (HIV) is a viral
STD,ie, Viral Sexually Transmitted Diseases that
damages the body's immune system, making it
unable to fight infection. HIV causes AIDS (Acquired
Immunodeficiency Syndrome), for which there is no
cure.

(A) <u>Symptoms And Signs Of HIV In Men Women And Children</u>:

There are many people suffering with <u>HIV</u> who
do not just know that actually they are the infected
person. In whole United States it is very less likely
that the 20% of the HIV-positive individual are simply
unaware of the fact that they are infected.

There are also many people who do not just develop
symptom after they first getting the infection with the

HIV. There are others as well who has the history of the flulike problems or illness in several days to the weeks after the exposure to the virus. The early HIV symptoms do also include the fever, tiredness, headache, and the enlarged lymph of the nodes in neck. The symptoms do usually disappear on the own in few weeks. However after that there are also few person that feel normal and also might have no symptoms at all. This is an asymptomatic phase, which is often last for one or more years.

The simple progression of the disease is that it varies widely between the individual. This state may last from a few months to sometime for more than the time of 10 years. During the large period virus of HIV continues to get multiplied with the active and then also infects and kill to all the cell of immune system. The virus can also destroy cells which are known to be primary infection fighters, which are a type of the white blood cell that is also called the CD4 cells.

AIDS is supposed to be a later state of the HIV infection. This is supposed to be done whenever the body starts losing the ability of fighting the simple infections. Once CD4 cell count goes low enough then the infected people is said to be with the AIDS. Sometime the diagnosis process of AIDS is also made because of the fact that the person had unusual infection or the cancers that shows that how weak immune system is.

The infection that does happen with the AIDS is called the opportunistic infections. The infection that include but they are not only limited to it are:

a. Pneupneumonia, which is caused by the Pneumocystis that causes wheezing;

b. Brain infection along with toxoplasmosis that cause trouble in thinking

c. Widespread infection of a bacteria known as MAC (Mycobacterium Avium Complex)

d. Yeast infection of swallowing tube.

e. Widespread diseases along with certain types of fungi like the histoplasmosis

(B) How it spreads?:

The HIV can be transmitted whenever the virus of HIV enters to the body . It is usually done by injecting the infected cells or the semen. There are also several others possible ways through which this HIV virus can easily enter in the human body. The major ways of them are as follows:

a. The very common cause of the occurrence of the HIV AIDS is the sex which is done with a partner who does already have the HIV virus in his body.

b. Sometimes the HIV virus can also enter in the body of some of the person through the HIV infected injections.

c. It sometime can also be transferred to babies by women when they give birth to the child

d. Sometime in setting the health care unwanted needles get in the body and they causes the HIV virus to get in the body of the person and hence HIV occurs to him.

(C) Early Signs and Test Of HIV:

The early signs are supposed to be the indicator that exactly when the help of a medical practitioner is supposed to be taken. The early signs in some of the cases are so simple that people ignore that they might be having suffering from the problems of HIV AIDS. This is the main reason that why there are lakhs of people in this world who are living with the infection of HIV AIDS that is the HIV virus is active in their bodies. Fever is the very basic symptom of any problem and this is also caused by the HIV virus after a week or two of time you get the virus in your body. This is why the diagnostic tests can play the major role in it.

HIV infection commonly diagnosed with the blood test. There are also three main types of the tests which are also very commonly used: HIV antibody test, RNA test and the combination test that can detect both the antibodies and the piece of a virus which is called p24 protein. Additionally the blood test which is known as western blot can also be used in order to confirm diagnosis.

No test supposed to be perfect because it may sometime also be falsely negative or falsely positive. This is why the testing for the HIV usually known to be the Two Steps process. If it comes out to be positive then it is positive and the second test is done in order to confirm this result. The antibody tests are known as the common initial test used for HIV. There are other different types of the antibody tests also available.

(D) Treatment of HIV:

Over to the last few years several drugs has become commonly available to cure for both the infection of HIV and the associated infection such as cancer. These are the drugs which are also called a highly active and antiretroviral therapy (HAART) that have the substantially reduced complications of HIV and of deaths. Still the medications do not supposed to cure the HIV/AIDS. In a case the patient was being treated for the cancer and apparently he got cured of the HIV through the use of the stem cell transplant. However this is not usually recommended to cure the HIV AIDS due to risk of the mortality and the uncertain chances of the success.

HIV/AIDS at a Glance:
- HIV is the infection that causes AIDS.
- HIV has few or no symptoms for up to 10 years or more before symptoms of AIDS develop.
- There is no cure for HIV/AIDS, but treatment is available.
- HIV can be spread during sex play.
- Latex and female condoms offer very good protection against HIV.

2. Genital Herpes:

Genital herpes is caused by the herpes simplex virus and is interchangeable with Type I herpes, which causes cold sores around the mouth and face. Having oral sex or intercourse with someone infected by either type of herpes can spread the disease. Genital herpes causes an outbreak of painful blisters. The virus then goes dormant, but cannot be completely eliminated.

Genital Herpes at a Glance:
- A very common sexually transmitted disease (STD)
- Can affect the mouth (oral herpes) or genitals (genital herpes)
- Easily spread with or without symptoms
- Treatment available for herpes symptoms
- There are ways to reduce your risk of getting herpes

3. HPV and Genital Warts

Genital human papillomavirus (HPV) is a common STD that can cause genital warts and increase the risk of cervical cancer. There is a campaign in the medical community to have teen-age girls vaccinated against HPV to cut the spread of genital HPV through sexual contact.

HPV and Genital Warts at a Glance:
- A common sexually transmitted disease (STD)
- Spread easily by skin-to-skin contact
- Treatment available for genital warts symptoms
- There are ways to reduce your risk of getting genital warts

4. Hepatitis:

Hepatitis is a virus that causes inflammation of the liver and can lead to liver diseases. Hepatitis B, which can cause jaundice, fatigue, vomiting and fever, can be transmitted through sexual contact. Most hepatitis B sufferers recover with anti-viral drug therapy, but some become chronic carriers and are infectious for life.

Hepatitis B at a Glance:
- A kind of liver infection
- Often has no symptoms

- No cure, but the infection often goes away on its own
- Many states require the hepatitis B vaccine for <u>school</u> children
- Can be spread during sex play
- Easily spread with or without symptoms
- Condoms offer good protection for people not vaccinated

(B). <u>Bacterial Sexually Transmitted Diseases</u>:

1. <u>Syphilis</u>:

Syphilis first shows up as a painless sore in the area of sexual contact. Some time later the disease will move into a highly infectious stage with a spotty rash on the chest, face, palms or soles of the feet. If left untreated, syphilis can damage the central nervous system and the brain.

<u>Syphilis at a Glance</u>:
- A sexually transmitted disease (STD)
- Often has no symptoms
- Treatment available in the early stages
- Condoms offer good protection

2. Gonorrhea:

Gonorrhea is transmitted through vaginal, oral or anal sex. It can successfully be treated with antibiotics, but if left untreated can cause pelvic pain, vaginal discharge and pelvic inflammatory disease.

Gonorrhea at a Glance:
- A common sexually transmitted disease (STD)
- Often has no symptoms
- Easily treated
- Easily spread with or without symptoms
- Condoms offer good protection

3. Chancroid:

Chancroid is a sexually transmitted disease caused by a bacterium. It is common in tropical countries.

Chancroid at a Glance:
- A sexually transmitted disease (STD)
- Common symptoms include sores on the genitals
- Treatment is available
- Easily spread
- Condoms reduce your risk of infection

4. <u>Chlamydia</u>:

Chlamydia trachomatis, known simply as Chlamydia, is spread through vaginal, anal or oral sex. If not diagnosed in early stages and treated with antibiotics, Chlamydia can spread and cause pelvic inflammatory disease, which can lead to ectopic pregnancies and infertility.

<u>Chlamydia at a Glance</u>:
- A common sexually transmitted disease (STD)
- Often has no symptoms
- Easily treated
- Easily spread with or without symptoms.
- Condoms offer good protection

5. <u>PID</u>:

Pelvic inflammatory disease (PID) occurs when bacteria move from the vagina or cervix into the uterus, fallopian tubes, ovaries, or pelvis. Most cases of PID are due to the bacteria that cause <u>chlamydia</u> and <u>gonorrhea</u>. These are sexually transmitted infections (STIs). The most common way a woman develops PID is by having unprotected sex with someone who has a sexually transmitted infection.

PID at a Glance
- PID stands for pelvic inflammatory disease
- Common and serious complication of some sexually transmitted diseases (STDs)
- Often, there are no symptoms
- Condoms reduce your risk

6. Trichomoniasis:

Trichomoniasis is causes by a small parasite that is usually sexually transmitted. Symptoms include a frothy vaginal discharge. Trichomoniasis can be treated with oral antibiotics or vaginal cream

Trichomoniasis at a Glance:
- Often called "trich"
- A sexually transmitted infection
- Often has no symptoms
- Easily treated
- Condoms reduce your risk of infection

Safer Sex (Safe Sex) at a Glance:

- Reduces our risk of getting a sexually transmitted disease (STD)
- Using condoms makes vaginal or anal intercourse safer sex
- Using condoms or other barriers makes oral sex safer sex

- Having sex play without intercourse can be even safer sex
- Safer sex can be very pleasurable and exciting